# Sensei Self Development

## Mental Health Chronicles Series

*Strategies to Joy*

Sensei Paul David

# Copyright Page

Sensei Self Development -
Strategies to Joy,
by Sensei Paul David
Copyright © 2024

All rights reserved.

978-1-77848-299-1
SSD_Journals_Amazon_PaperbackBook_
Strategies to Joy

978-1-77848-298-4 SSD_Journals_Amazon_eBook_
Strategies to Joy

978-1-77848-436-0
SSD_Journals_Ingram_Paperback_
Strategies to Joy

This book is not authorized for free distribution copying.

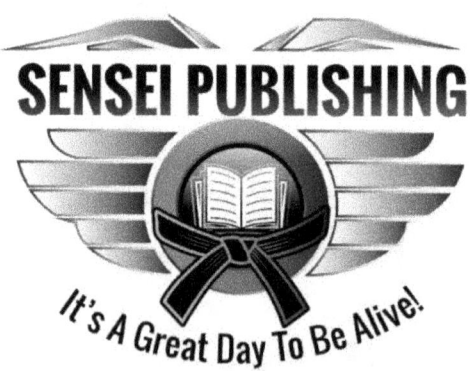

www.senseipublishing.com

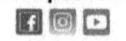

@senseipublishing
#senseipublishing

# Get/Share Your FREE SSD Mental Health Chronicles at www.senseiselfdevelopment.care

or

## CLICK HERE

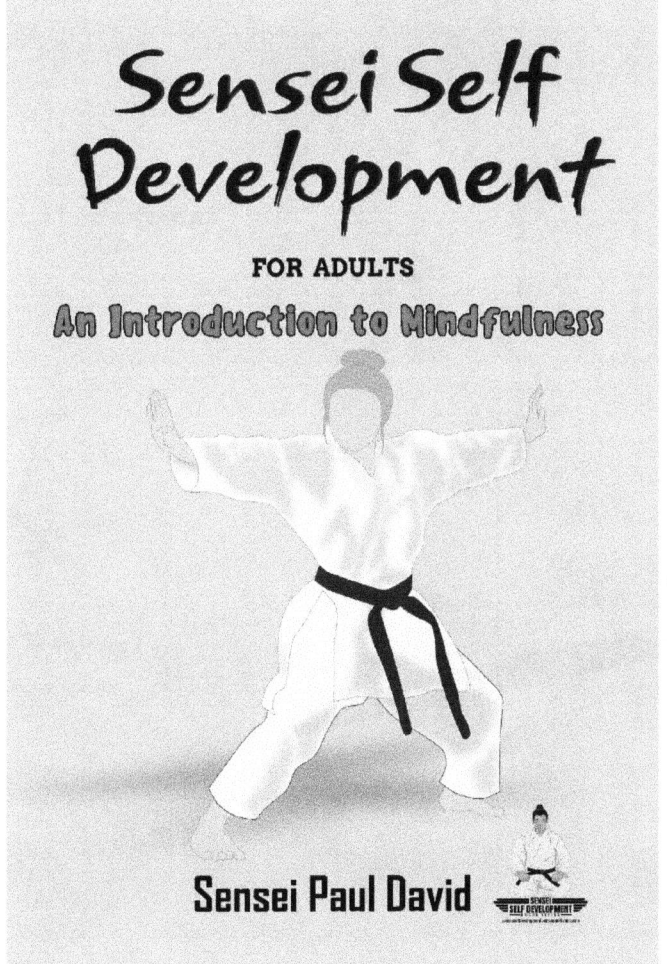

# Check Out The SSD Chronicles Series CLICK HERE

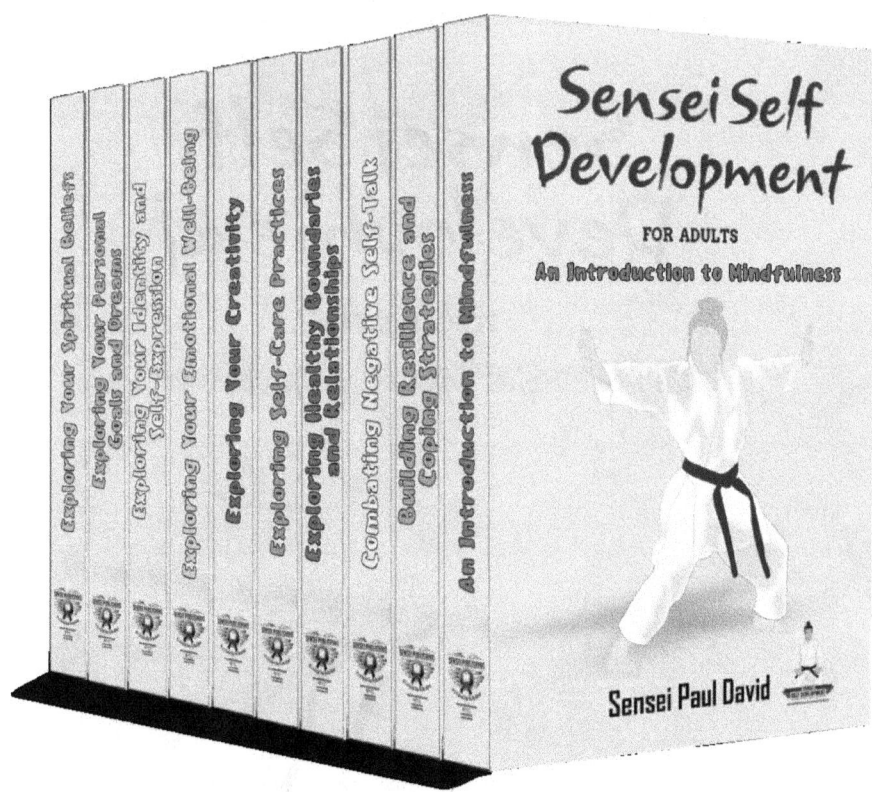

# Dedication

To those who courageously take action towards self-improvement - you are helping to evolve the world for generations to come.

- It's a great day to be alive!

**If Found Please Contact:**

_____


**Reward If Found:**

_____

# MY COMMITMENT

I, _____ commit to writing This Sensei Self Development Journal for at least 10 days in a row, starting: _____

Writing this journal is valuable to me because:

_____

_____

_____

_____

_____

If I finish a minimum of 10 consecutive days of writing in this journal, I will reward myself by:

_____

_____

_____

_____

_____

_____

If I don't finish 10 days of writing this journal, I will promise to:

_____

_____

_____

_____

_____

I will do the following things to ensure that I write in my Sensei Self Development Journal every day:

_____

_____

_____

_____

_____

# Get/Share Your FREE All-Ages Mental Health eBook Now at
## www.senseiselfdevelopment.com
## Or CLICK HERE

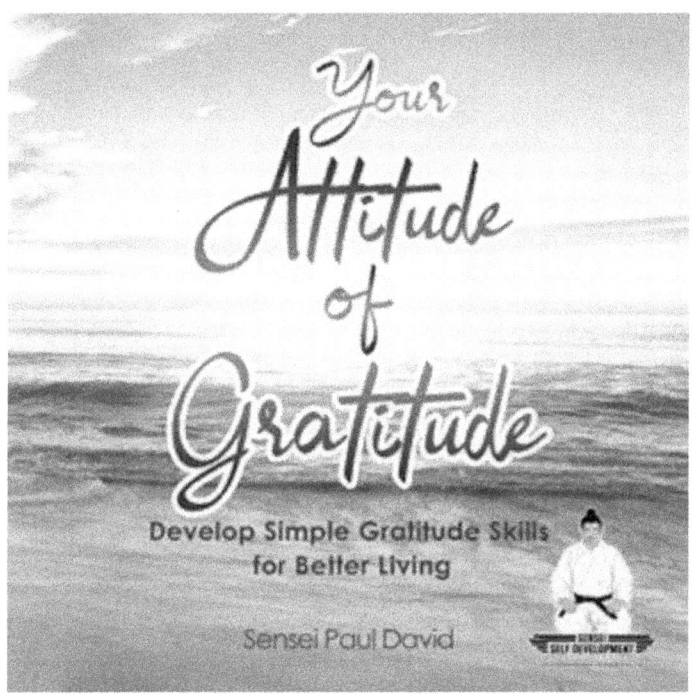

senseiselfdevelopment.com

# Check Out Another Book In The SSD BOOK SERIES:
senseipublishing.com/SSD_SERIES
## CLICK HERE

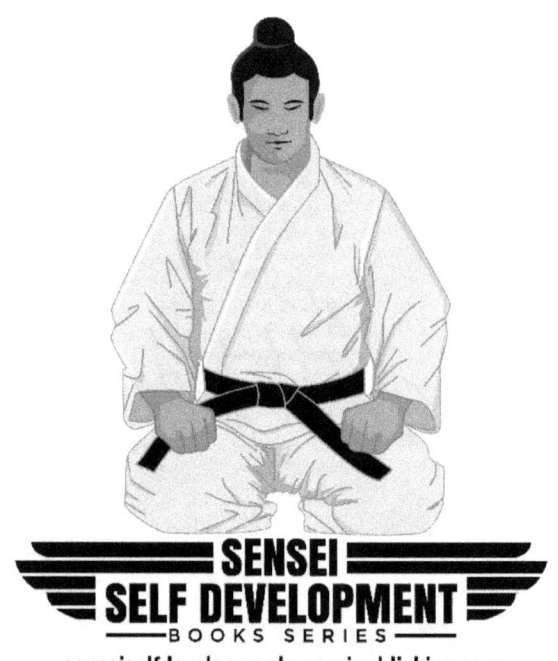

# Join Our Publishing Journey!

If you would like to receive FUTURE FREE BOOKS and get to know us better, please click www.senseipublishing.com and join our newsletter by entering your email address in the pop-up box.

**Follow Our Blog: senseipauldavid.ca**

Follow/Like/Subscribe: Facebook, Instagram, YouTube: @senseipublishing

Scan the QR Code with your phone or tablet
to follow us on social media: Like / Subscribe / Follow

# A Message From The Author:
## Sensei Paul David

Dear Reader,

Welcome to the world of mental health journaling – a sacred space for self-reflection, growth, and healing. Within these pages, you hold the power to uplift your spirit, invigorate your mind, and nourish your goals.

In a world that often moves at blink-and-you'll-miss-it speed, it's crucial to make time for self-care and self-discovery.

Anxiety, stress, and emotional turbulence may have clouded your mind, making it difficult to find clarity and peace within. But fear not! Together, we will navigate the labyrinth of emotions, and experiences, helping to simplify the path to mental well-being.

This journal is not merely a bunch of blank pages awaiting your words. It is your compassionate companion, offering solace and understanding during your unique journey. Here, you are free to unburden yourself, celebrate small and large victories, and confront the challenges that may still linger.

Within the sheltered realm of these pages, there is no judgment, no expectation, and no pressure. Your unique experience and perspective hold immeasurable worth, and your voice deserves to be heard. Whether you choose to fill the lines with eloquence or simply scribble fragments of your thoughts, please remember each entry is a valuable contribution to your growth.

In this sacred space, you are challenged to take off the mask we so often wear in the outside world. It is here that you can be raw, vulnerable, and authentic – allowing your true self to be seen and embraced without reservation. By giving yourself permission to explore the depths of your emotions and confront the shadows that may lurk within, you will discover profound insights and find the healing you seek over time.

As you embark on this journaling journey, I encourage you to embrace the process itself rather than fixate solely on the outcome. Remember, it is not about reaching a certain destination or ticking off boxes on a list of accomplishments. Rather, it is about cultivating self-awareness, fostering self-compassion, and nurturing a sense of curiosity about the intricate workings of your intelligently beautiful mind.

In the quiet moments of reflection, let your pen become a bridge between your inner world and the possibilities that lie ahead. Create a sanctuary for your thoughts, fears, triumphs, and dreams. As you pour your heart onto these pages, allow your words to be a living testament to courage, resilience, and an unwavering commitment to your own well-being.

I am honored to be a part of your journey, and I believe in your ability to navigate the twists and turns with grace and resilience. Remember, you are not alone in this – countless others have walked similar paths, faced similar challenges, and emerged stronger and wiser on the other side. You have the power to reclaim all of your untapped joy, cultivate a positive mindset that serves you, and foster a deep sense of self-love and peaceful confident. – And it will take a worth effort and time.

So, open the first page of this journal with hope, curiosity, and an open heart and open mind. Embrace the transformative power of self-reflection, and allow it to guide you towards a life of greater fulfilment and peace. Each journaling session is an opportunity to not only connect with yourself but also to rekindle the light within that sometimes flickers but never extinguishes.

Remember, the pages you are about to fill are not just a record of your journey but also a testament to your strength, resilience, and indomitable spirit. Cherish this space, invest in yourself, and let your words be an ode to the magnificent journey of becoming whole.

With great respect for your decision to evolve,

Paul

# MY CONVICTION

*Please circle your answers below*

I am DECIDING to be patient with myself and this PROCESS each time I journal toward my improved state of mental well-being

YES     NO

"The present moment is filled with joy and happiness. If you are attentive, you will see it."

*Thich Nhat Hanh*

# Introduction

Past few years have been challenging for nearly everyone, and it's understandable if you're finding it harder to feel positive and joyful. In fact, a recent survey shows that happiness in America has reached its lowest point in fifty years.

The good news is that, although happiness is partly determined by genetics and the fulfillment of basic needs like safety, shelter, and food, there's a significant portion you can influence. Small, consistent actions focused on the positives in life can, over time, become ingrained habits that significantly boost your happiness.

Additionally, increasing the amount of joy in your daily life can also improve your overall well-being. Happiness consists of two aspects: life satisfaction, which is the sense that things are going well in your life, and the experience of frequent positive emotions such as pride, curiosity, enthusiasm, tranquility, and joy.

Here are the top evidence-based strategies for discovering more joy in various aspects of your life - in your work and job, at home, and in your everyday activities - beginning right now.

## Create a Joy List

To create a Joy List, start by pondering what genuinely brings you happiness. This could range from being with friends, to nature walks, to the scent of flowers. Reflect on your past joyful moments to find inspiration. Once you have your list, actively seek out these experiences to enhance your joy.

Here are some examples from my own Joy List:

1. Hearing a song that reminds me of my childhood.

2. Enjoying that first sip of coffee in the morning.

3. Finishing a really good book.

4. Being in my warm bed while it's pouring rain outside.

5. When someone tells me 'Let me know when you're home safe.'

6. Finding a piece of clothing that fits just right.

7. The smell of freshly cut grass.

8. Looking up at clear blue skies.

9. Watching the beauty of a sunset or sunrise.

10. The crisp crunch of fall leaves under my feet.

11. Looking back at the room after I have just finished cleaning it up.

12. Walking on the beach.

Recognizing the small things that bring joy can make you more inclined to seek them out and appreciate them deeply.

Often, we're lost in our thoughts, but being conscious of joy-bringing elements around us brings our focus back to the present, enhancing our experience of joy. Have you experienced this? For instance, sinking into warm bath water after a stressful day and suddenly realizing how soothing it feels. Compare this to times when you're in the same warm, comforting water but too distracted to notice, hastily getting out without truly savoring the moment, which brings me to our next strategy.

## Savoring

Imagine going on a vacation to Hawaii or dining at an upscale restaurant you've always wanted to visit. Such moments are undoubtedly memorable. Yet, there's also joy in the everyday. Finding a beautiful, secluded spot in a park, watching a breathtaking sunset, or the simple act of reading a book in a cozy corner can be deeply satisfying. Even routine activities, like a family game night or attending community events, can become extraordinary if you pause to appreciate them.

Savoring not only creates positive feelings, but it also strengthens and extends them. In a study, participants kept diaries over a month, recording their positive activities and how much they savored these moments. The results showed that those who savored their experiences a lot maintained a high level of happiness, regardless of the rest of their day. On the other hand, those who savored less needed many positive events to feel similarly happy.

So, don't forget to pause and smell the roses.

There is joy in that.

## Embrace Awe as Much as Possible

In recent years, there's been a growing interest in how feelings of awe contribute to happiness and good health. A project, known as "Project Awe," was initiated by a university in California in 2013 to explore this. A study published in 2015 found that college students who frequently experienced positive emotions, particularly awe, had lower levels of interleukin-6, an inflammation indicator.

Furthermore, awe might even enhance our generosity and ethical decision-making. A 2015 study across five experiments found that feelings of awe led people to be more generous and considerate of what's beneficial for the community.

Experiencing awe doesn't require grand events. Simple activities like a walk around the block can evoke this feeling. Allen Klein, an author, suggests going on an "awe walk" where you temporarily set aside your mental to-do list and instead focus on the wonder in the small things around you. This approach can be a simple yet effective way to incorporate a sense of awe into daily life.

Here is a list of things you can do to induce awe:

1. Watching a captivating documentary about the mysteries of space and the cosmos.
2. Observing the beauty of a blooming flower in your garden.
3. Stargazing on a clear night and contemplating the vastness of the universe.
4. Exploring a science museum and learning about the wonders of our world.
5. Listening to a thunderstorm's powerful rumble and witnessing lightning.
6. Reading about the incredible diversity of life in the depths of the ocean.
7. Taking a nature walk and encountering unexpected wildlife.

## Look at the Bright Side of Things

Optimism partly comes from your genes, but it's also a learned trait. Even if you come from a family of pessimists, you can still develop a more optimistic outlook. Optimism isn't about denying the difficulties of a situation. For instance, in the face of job loss, instead of succumbing to thoughts like, "I'll never recover from this," an optimist would view it as a challenging yet hopeful opportunity, thinking, "This is hard, but it's a chance to reassess my career goals and find work that really brings me joy."

Positive thinking and surrounding yourself with optimistic people can make a significant difference. Optimism, just like pessimism, is contagious. Therefore, it's beneficial to associate with those who have a positive and hopeful perspective on life.

## Be Generous

The saying "It's better to give than to receive" is popular for a reason. It holds a lot of truth, especially when it comes to fostering joy.

Research involving surveys from 200,000 adults across the globe found that people who donated to charity were generally happier than those who didn't, regardless of their financial situation. This happiness boost might be because giving activates brain areas linked to pleasure, social connection, and trust.

Even if you're on a budget, the act of giving, no matter how small, can significantly impact your happiness. In an experiment, students were given small amounts of money and instructed to spend it on themselves or others by the end of the day. The findings were clear: those who spent the money on others felt happier than those who spent it on themselves, and the amount – whether $5 or $20 – didn't make a difference.

What's crucial then? It's where and how you give. The joy of giving is heightened when you can see the impact of your contribution and feel a connection to the people or cause you're supporting. And if financial giving isn't an option, the same benefits can be obtained through acts of kindness, like making a thoughtful phone call to someone in need.

## Spend Time in Nature

Imagine yourself in the heart of a tranquil forest at dawn. The world around you is just waking up, bathed in the soft glow of the early morning sun. You are surrounded by tall, majestic trees, their leaves whispering secrets in the gentle breeze. The air is crisp and cool, filled with the fresh scent of pine and earth. As you walk along the forest path, the soft moss beneath your feet cushions your steps. Birds sing a melodious welcome to the new day, and a distant stream murmurs a soothing lullaby. The peace of the forest envelops you, calming your mind and rejuvenating your spirit. In this moment, you are part of nature's quiet awakening.

There's a wealth of evidence showing that time spent in nature is beneficial for your well-being. Walking along tranquil, tree-filled paths can lead to significant improvements in mental health and even alter brain activity. Those who walk in natural settings tend to have "quieter" brains, with brain scans indicating less blood flow to areas associated with repetitive thought or rumination. Additionally, studies suggest that even viewing images of nature can uplift your mood.

The impact of sunlight is also noteworthy. Seasonal affective disorder, a type of depression related to changes in seasons, is a recognized condition with varying prevalence across different regions, from around 1.4 percent in sunnier areas to 9.7 percent in less sunny ones. Exposure to natural sunlight, either by spending time outdoors or being in a space with ample natural light, is known to positively influence mood.

## Get Active

It turns out that simply getting up and moving can make you happier. A study involving cellphone users' movement and mood found that people felt happiest when they had been moving in the last 15 minutes, compared to when they were sitting or lying down. Most of the time, the activity that boosted mood wasn't intense exercise, but just gentle walking. While it's not certain if being active makes you happier or if happy people are more active, there's a clear relationship between being more physically active and experiencing greater happiness and health.

## Practice Gratitude

Embracing gratitude involves recognizing and appreciating the positive aspects of life, both big and small. It's about acknowledging the good in our lives, which can often go overlooked amidst daily challenges and routines. Practicing gratitude can lead to a range of benefits, including improved mood, greater optimism, and enhanced overall well-being.

One effective way to cultivate gratitude is through maintaining a gratitude journal. This involves regularly writing down things you are thankful for. It could be as simple as a sunny day, a good meal, or a kind gesture from a stranger. By doing this, you shift your focus from what's missing in your life to the abundance that exists within it.

Another approach is expressing gratitude to others. This could be through a heartfelt thank you, a thoughtful note, or even a small gift to show appreciation. Such acts of gratitude not only make others feel valued but also reinforce your own feelings of thankfulness.

Incorporating gratitude into your daily routine need not be time-consuming or complicated. It can be as straightforward as taking a moment each day to reflect on something you're grateful for, or expressing appreciation to someone who's made a difference in your life. Over time, this practice can transform your perspective, making you more aware of the good that surrounds you and enriching your experience of life.

## Declutter (But Keep What Brings You Joy)

Organizing your space is good for your mind and body. It helps prevent accidents, keeps things hygienic, and makes it easier to find important items.

Excessive clutter can be a sign of deeper issues. People dealing with emotional trauma, brain injuries, or mental health challenges like attention deficit disorder, depression, or grief often struggle with keeping their space organized. In extreme cases, this leads to hoarding, which some experts consider a mental illness, although it's not officially recognized as such.

Most people aren't hoarders but can still benefit from understanding this extreme. Being chronically disorganized can impact your emotional, physical, or social health.

Change is possible with therapy or guidance from self-help books. Happiness experts advise keeping things that are meaningful, like a child's drawing or a family heirloom, and getting rid of the rest.

Decluttering tips include:

- Folding items neatly.

- Keeping only what makes you truly happy.

- Throwing away unnecessary papers.

- Sorting through all your clothes, keeping only those you use and love.

- Organizing your closet by color.

- If you tend to hold onto things for sentimental reasons, choose one item from each collection or the collection with the best memories.

- Instead of buying souvenirs on vacation, take a photo.

- Focus on experiences, not material things.

- For children's school projects, take photos and keep only a few significant items each year.

This approach helps create a space that's not only tidier but also more meaningful, filled with items that truly matter to you.

## The Joy Movements

Exercise, even in small amounts, is widely known to lift your mood, a phenomenon often referred to as the 'feel-better effect'. Any form of physical activity, be it a stroll, a swim, or a yoga session, can elevate your emotions, but there are certain movements that are especially effective in generating joy.

Studies across various cultures have pinpointed movements typically associated with the expression of joy: raising your arms high, swaying side to side as one might do while enjoying music, rhythmic motions like bouncing to a beat, or expansive movements such as spinning with arms wide open. These actions don't just convey joy; research indicates they can actually provoke these feelings.

In several small-scale studies, participants who engaged in these types of movements reported feeling more positive emotions. Conversely, motions that involved collapsing or constricting the body were linked to negative emotions like sadness and fear. Interestingly, another study found that these 'joy movements' have an amplified effect when you see others performing them too, possibly because happiness is known to be infectious.

## The 1-Minute Rule for Happiness

Complete any task that can be done in under a minute.


Here's a list you can try:


- Hang up a coat.

- Respond to an email.

- Place a dish in the dishwasher.

-Straighten a stack of books. Put away any loose items on your desk.

-Throw dirty clothes into the laundry basket.

-Fluff a pillow on the couch.

-Set up your coffee maker for the next morning


Implementing the one-minute rule in your daily routine can offer a quick sense of achievement and productivity, bringing a burst of happiness from accomplishing so much in such a short time. As an added benefit, you'll end up with a tidier space, contributing further to your sense of well-being.

## Spend Time with Happy People

There's compelling evidence that our happiness is intertwined with the happiness of those around us. Insight into this comes from the Framingham Heart Study, a long-term project begun in 1948 that has followed three generations. Originally aimed at identifying heart disease risk factors, it has amassed extensive data on health, diet, exercise, stress, family dynamics, and happiness.

In assessing happiness, participants were asked about their feelings over the past week, including hopefulness about the future, enjoyment of life, and feelings of equality with others.

Yale researchers delved into this data to examine happiness and social connections.

The study's design enabled them to observe changes in happiness over time and, importantly, track the participants' social networks, including family, friends, and colleagues.

The analysis led to several key findings:

- An individual's happiness is influenced by the happiness of those they are connected with.
- Happy and unhappy people tend to cluster in social networks.
- A person's happiness can have an impact up to three degrees of separation, affecting their friends, their friends' friends, and even extending to the friends of those friends.
- People surrounded by many happy individuals are more likely to become happier in the future.

- Having an additional happy friend can increase your own likelihood of being happy by about 9 percent.
- Proximity matters; being physically closer to happy friends and family can boost your own happiness.

These findings underscore the significance of the company we keep and how our social environment can shape our personal happiness.

## Volunteer

Volunteering offers not just emotional satisfaction but also tangible health benefits like reduced blood pressure and a lower mortality rate. It's known to strengthen resilience, enhancing your ability to recover from various challenges, whether they're minor setbacks or major traumas.

A comprehensive study by the University of Exeter concluded that volunteering is almost like a happiness prescription that can extend and improve the quality of life. This conclusion came after reviewing 40 studies on volunteering, which collectively indicated that volunteers experience less depression, increased life satisfaction, and overall well-being. Notably, in five extensive studies on volunteerism, participants had a 22% lower mortality rate over the study period.

While it could be argued that naturally happier people might be more inclined to volunteer, the overall evidence strongly suggests a significant connection between giving time to others and personal happiness.

## Use Breathing Excercise

As you engage in deep breathing, a sense of tranquility begins to wash over you. Each deliberate, slow inhalation feels like a gentle wave smoothing the rough edges of your mind. Your muscles, which may have been tensed up under the day's burdens, start to loosen and relax as if they are finally being given permission to let go of their constant vigilance.

With every exhale, there's an unspoken release of worries that you might not have even realized you were holding onto. It's as if with each breath out, a bit of stress and anxiety is being expelled, leaving your body lighter and more serene. The rhythm of your breathing becomes a subtle, yet powerful anchor, keeping you moored in the present moment.

This simple act of drawing in air deeply, filling your lungs, and then releasing it, becomes a profound exercise in mindfulness. You become acutely aware of the here and now - the sensation of air passing through your nostrils, the gentle rise and fall of your chest, the way your body instinctively knows how to relax and unwind with this age-old technique. It's a moment of connection between mind, body, and breath, a quiet reminder of the simple, yet powerful tools we possess to bring ourselves back to a state of calm and balance.

There is a lightness of being in breathing, what we call joy.

Recent scientific research is beginning to validate the age-old benefits of controlled breathing. Studies suggest that specific breathing techniques can significantly reduce symptoms of various conditions including anxiety, insomnia, PTSD, depression, and attention deficit disorder. Historically, breath control has been an integral part of yoga, known as pranayama, used to enhance concentration and vitality. Additionally, it has deep roots in spiritual practices, such as Buddhism, where breath-meditation is a key technique for achieving enlightenment.

Here's a simple breathing exercise you can try:

4-7-8 Breathing Technique:

- Inhale through your nose quietly for a count of 4.

- Hold your breath for a count of 7.

- Exhale completely through your mouth, making a whoosh sound, for a count of 8.

- Repeat this cycle for four breaths.

## Eliminate What Drains Your Joy.

I remember a conversation with a friend who's savvy in finance. He said something that stuck with me: in investing, it's not just about how to make money, but also about how to avoid losing it.

This principle applies broadly. Take health, for instance. Instead of only focusing on what you can do to become healthier, it's equally important to consider what's currently detrimental to your health.

The same goes for happiness. While it's crucial to engage in activities that make us happy, it's equally vital to steer clear of those that sap our joy and bring us down.

So, let's look at some typical joy-drainers that you might want to cut back on or remove from your life:

1. Negative Self-Talk: The way you talk to yourself has a profound impact on your well-being. Constant self-criticism and pessimism can drain your joy. Work on replacing negative thoughts with positive affirmations.

2. Toxic Relationships: People who consistently bring negativity or drama into your life can deplete your emotional energy. It's important to set boundaries or distance yourself from such relationships.

3. Overcommitting: Spreading yourself too thin can lead to burnout and resentment. Learn to say no to tasks or commitments that don't align with your priorities or bring you joy.

4. Dwelling on the Past: Constantly revisiting past mistakes or unpleasant events can trap you in a cycle of regret and sadness. Focus on the present and what you can control.

5. Excessive Worrying: Worrying about things beyond your control can create unnecessary stress. Practice mindfulness to stay grounded in the present moment.

6. Comparing Yourself to Others: This can lead to feelings of inadequacy and jealousy. Remember that everyone's journey is unique, and focus on your own growth and achievements.

7. Mindless Consumption: Whether it's social media, news, or TV, consuming content that doesn't enrich your life can be a major time and joy waster. Be selective about what you consume.

8. Neglecting Self-Care: Not taking care of your physical, emotional, and mental health can leave you feeling depleted. Regular self-care is crucial for maintaining your joy.

9. Clutter and Disorganization: A cluttered space can lead to a cluttered mind. Keeping your living and working spaces tidy and organized can help maintain a sense of calm and joy.

10. Perfectionism: Striving for perfection sets an unattainable standard that can lead to disappointment. Embrace imperfection and give yourself grace.

Identifying and addressing these aspects of your life can help create more space for joy and fulfillment. Remember, it's a process and involves making conscious choices every day.

Before We Get Started...

Remember, mindfulness journaling is a personal practice, and these questions are meant to guide and inspire you. Feel free to adapt and modify them to suit your needs and preferences. Explore, reflect, and embrace the opportunity to deepen your self-awareness and cultivate a sense of inner peace.

Date ___/___/___ : S  M  T  W  Th  F  S

**I feel:**
(please circle)

😊 because _____
😁 because _____
😋 because _____
😟 because _____
😠 because _____

### Today I Am Grateful For
1. _____
2. _____
3. _____

What could help transform today into a remarkable day?

### Reflective Writing

What is the most joyful project you have undertaken recently?

_____
_____
_____
_____
_____
_____
_____

**What is a simple way to add joy to your daily routine?**

A) Taking a walk in nature
B) Watching a movie
C) Checking social media
D) Eating a large meal

All Are Correct - Choose The Response You Feel Is Most Important To Remember

Date ___/___/___ : S  M  T  W  Th  F  S

I feel:
(please circle)

because _____  because _____  because _____  because _____  because _____

## Today I Am Grateful For

1. _____
2. _____
3. _____

What could help transform today into a remarkable day?

## Reflective Writing

What was the biggest challenge you faced when engaging in joyful endeavours?

_____
_____
_____
_____
_____
_____
_____

**How can you cultivate gratitude in your life?**

A) Writing thank you notes
B) Complaining to friends
C) Watching the news
D) Checking your phone constantly

All Are Correct - Choose The Response You Feel Is Most Important To Remember

Date ___/___/___ : S  M  T  W  Th  F  S

**I feel:**
(please circle)

😊 because _____
😁 because _____
😋 because _____
😟 because _____
😠 because _____

### Today I Am Grateful For
1. _____
2. _____
3. _____

What could help transform today into a remarkable day?

## Reflective Writing
What do you do to keep your happiness flowing?

_____
_____
_____
_____
_____
_____
_____
_____

**What is a helpful strategy for dealing with negative thoughts?**

A) Ignoring them
B) Sharing them on social media
C) Practicing positive self-talk
D) Dwelling on them

All Are Correct - Choose The Response You Feel Is Most Important To Remember

Date ___/___/___ : S  M  T  W  Th  F  S

**I feel:**
(please circle)

because _____  because _____  because _____  because _____  because _____

## Today I Am Grateful For
1. _____
2. _____
3. _____

What could help transform today into a remarkable day?
_____

### Reflective Writing
How have you learned to overcome your sadness?

_____
_____
_____
_____
_____
_____
_____
_____
_____

## How can you infuse joy into household chores?

A) Listening to music
B) Rushing through them
C) Multitasking
D) Avoiding them altogether

All Are Correct - Choose The Response You Feel Is Most Important To Remember

Date ___/___/___ : S  M  T  W  Th  F  S

**I feel:**
(please circle)

because _____  because _____  because _____  because _____  because _____

## Today I Am Grateful For

1. _____
2. _____
3. _____

What could help transform today into a remarkable day?

## Reflective Writing

What have been some of the successes you have experienced when being joyful?

_____
_____
_____
_____
_____
_____
_____

## What is a helpful tool for managing stress and promoting joy?

A) Meditation
B) Drinking alcohol
C) Overeating
D) Procrastinating

All Are Correct - Choose The Response You Feel Is Most Important To Remember

Date ___/___/___ : S  M  T  W  Th  F  S

**I feel:**
(please circle)

because _____   because _____   because _____   because _____   because _____

**Today I Am Grateful For**
1. _____
2. _____
3. _____

What could help transform today into a remarkable day?

**Reflective Writing**
What is your favorite joyful activity?

_____
_____
_____
_____
_____
_____
_____
_____

## How can you add spontaneity to your life?

A) Trying a new hobby
B) Sticking to a strict schedule
C) Avoiding new experiences
D) Setting rigid goals

All Are Correct - Choose The Response You Feel Is Most Important To Remember

Date ___/___/___ : S  M  T  W  Th  F  S

**I feel:**
(please circle)

because _____  because _____  because _____  because _____  because _____

### Today I Am Grateful For
1. _____
2. _____
3. _____

What could help transform today into a remarkable day?

## Reflective Writing
How has exploring your inner joyfulness impacted your life?

_____
_____
_____
_____
_____
_____
_____

**What is a key element of self-care that can increase joy?**

A) Neglecting your physical health
B) Setting unrealistic expectations
C) Prioritizing rest and relaxation
D) Focusing solely on work or school

All Are Correct - Choose The Response You Feel Is Most Important To Remember

Date ___ / ___ / ___ : S  M  T  W  Th  F  S

**I feel:**
(please circle)

because _____  because _____  because _____  because _____  because _____

## Today I Am Grateful For

1. _____
2. _____
3. _____

What could help transform today into a remarkable day?

## Reflective Writing

How do you handle criticism on your joyfulness?

_____
_____
_____
_____
_____
_____
_____
_____

## How can you foster meaningful connections with others?

A) Isolating yourself
B) Using social media as your primary source of communication
C) Actively listening and engaging with people
D) Gossiping about others

All Are Correct - Choose The Response You Feel Is Most Important To Remember

Date ___/___/___:  S   M   T   W   Th   F   S

**I feel:**
(please circle)

because _____  because _____  because _____  because _____  because _____

**Today I Am Grateful For**
1. _____
2. _____
3. _____

What could help transform today into a remarkable day?
_____

**Reflective Writing**

What are some of the most joyful ideas you have had?

_____
_____
_____
_____
_____
_____
_____
_____

## What is a helpful practice for managing emotions and promoting joy?

A) Suppressing your feelings
B) Expressing your emotions in a healthy way
C) Holding grudges and resentments
D) Avoiding difficult conversations

All Are Correct - Choose The Response You Feel Is Most Important To Remember

Date ___ / ___ / ___ : S  M  T  W  Th  F  S

**I feel:**
(please circle)

because _____  because _____  because _____  because _____  because _____

### Today I Am Grateful For
1. _____
2. _____
3. _____

What could help transform today into a remarkable day?

## Reflective Writing
How has exploring your joyfulness enabled you to become a better person?

_____
_____
_____
_____
_____
_____
_____

**How can setting boundaries improve your overall well-being and joy?**

A) Saying yes to everything
B) Allowing others to dictate your choices
C) Saying no when necessary
D) Overcommitting yourself

All Are Correct - Choose The Response You Feel Is Most Important To Remember

Date ___/___/___ : S  M  T  W  Th  F  S

**I feel:**
(please circle)

because _____   because _____   because _____   because _____   because _____

## Today I Am Grateful For

1. _____
2. _____
3. _____

What could help transform today into a remarkable day?

## Reflective Writing
What do you do when you feel sad?

_____
_____
_____
_____
_____
_____
_____
_____

**What is a simple way to practice mindfulness and increase joy?**

A) Worrying about the future
B) Dwelling on the past
C) Being fully present in the moment
D) Multitasking and trying to do many things at once

All Are Correct - Choose The Response You Feel Is Most Important To Remember

Date ___/___/___ : S  M  T  W  Th  F  S

**I feel:**
(please circle)

because _____  because _____  because _____  because _____  because _____

**Today I Am Grateful For**
1. _____
2. _____
3. _____

What could help transform today into a remarkable day?

**Reflective Writing**
How do you go about generating new and innovative ideas to make you happy?

_____
_____
_____
_____
_____
_____
_____
_____

## How can you incorporate more play into your life?

A) Avoiding fun activities
B) Prioritizing work and responsibilities
C) Trying new hobbies and activities
D) Overly planning and scheduling your free time

All Are Correct - Choose The Response You Feel Is Most Important To Remember

Date ___ / ___ / ___ : S  M  T  W  Th  F  S

**I feel:**
(please circle)

😊 because _____
😁 because _____
😋 because _____
😥 because _____
😠 because _____

### Today I Am Grateful For
1. _____
2. _____
3. _____

What could help transform today into a remarkable day?

### Reflective Writing
What techniques do you use to stay motivated when engaged in pursuit of happiness?

_____
_____
_____
_____
_____
_____
_____
_____

## Why is it important to celebrate small victories?

A) To constantly strive for perfection
B) To compare ourselves to others
C) To recognize our own growth and progress
D) To constantly criticize and judge ourselves

All Are Correct - Choose The Response You Feel Is Most Important To Remember

Date ___/___/___ : S  M  T  W  Th  F  S

I feel:
(please circle)

because _____  because _____  because _____  because _____  because _____

### Today I Am Grateful For
1. _____
2. _____
3. _____

What could help transform today into a remarkable day?

## Reflective Writing
What tips and tricks have you learned over the years that help you stay joyful?

_____
_____
_____
_____
_____
_____
_____

**What is a helpful strategy for overcoming perfectionism and increasing joy?**

A) Setting impossible standards for yourself
B) Comparing yourself to others
C) Practicing self-compassion and accepting imperfections
D) Avoiding challenges and risks

All Are Correct - Choose The Response You Feel Is Most Important To Remember

Date ___ / ___ / ___ : S  M  T  W  Th  F  S

**I feel:**
(please circle)

| 🙂 | 😁 | 😋 | 😟 | 😠 |
|---|---|---|---|---|
| because | because | because | because | because |
| _____ | _____ | _____ | _____ | _____ |

### Today I Am Grateful For
1. _____
2. _____
3. _____

What could help transform today into a remarkable day?
_____

### Reflective Writing
What do you feel is the biggest benefit of exploring your joyfulness?

_____
_____
_____
_____
_____
_____
_____
_____

## How can practicing self-care enhance joy in your life by?

A) taking time for yourself
B) practicing mindfulness
C) connecting with others
D) practicing gratitude, and treating yourself

All Are Correct - Choose The Response You Feel Is Most Important To Remember

As we reach the final pages of this journey through "Positive Mindset," I want to extend my heartfelt thanks to you. Your commitment to exploring positivity and its transformative power is not only commendable but a testament to your desire for personal growth and a richer, more fulfilling life experience.

Remember, the journey towards a positive mindset is ongoing and ever-evolving. Each day presents new opportunities to apply these principles, to learn, and to grow. I encourage you to revisit these pages whenever you need a reminder of your incredible potential to foster positivity and resilience in the face of life's challenges.

As we part ways, I leave you with a quote that has been a guiding star in my journey: "The greatest discovery of any generation is that a human can alter his life by altering his attitude."

– William James.

Thank you for allowing me to be a part of your journey. May your path be filled with light, hope, and endless possibilities. Farewell, and may you carry the spirit of positivity with you, today and always.

With gratitude and best wishes,

Sensei Paul David

# Reflective Writing

# The End

As you close the pages of this mindfulness journal, remember that each word you've written is a step on your journey towards self-awareness and inner peace. Embrace the moments of clarity, the revelations, and even the uncertainties you've encountered along the way. Let this journal be a testament to your growth and a reminder that every day offers a new opportunity to be present, to observe, and to appreciate the simple wonders of life. Carry these lessons forward, and may your path be filled with mindful moments and serene reflections. Until we meet again in these pages, be gentle with yourself and stay anchored in the now.

Mindfulness isn't difficult, we just need to remember to do it.

# Thank You!

If you found this book helpful, I would be grateful if you would **post an honest review on Amazon** so this book can reach other supportive readers like you!

All you need to do is digitally flip to the back and leave your review. Or visit amazon.com/author/senseipauldavid click the correct book cover and click on the blue link next to the yellow stars that say, "customer reviews."

## *As always...*
## *It's a great day to be alive!*

# Get/Share Your FREE SSD Mental Health Chronicles at www.senseiselfdevelopment.care

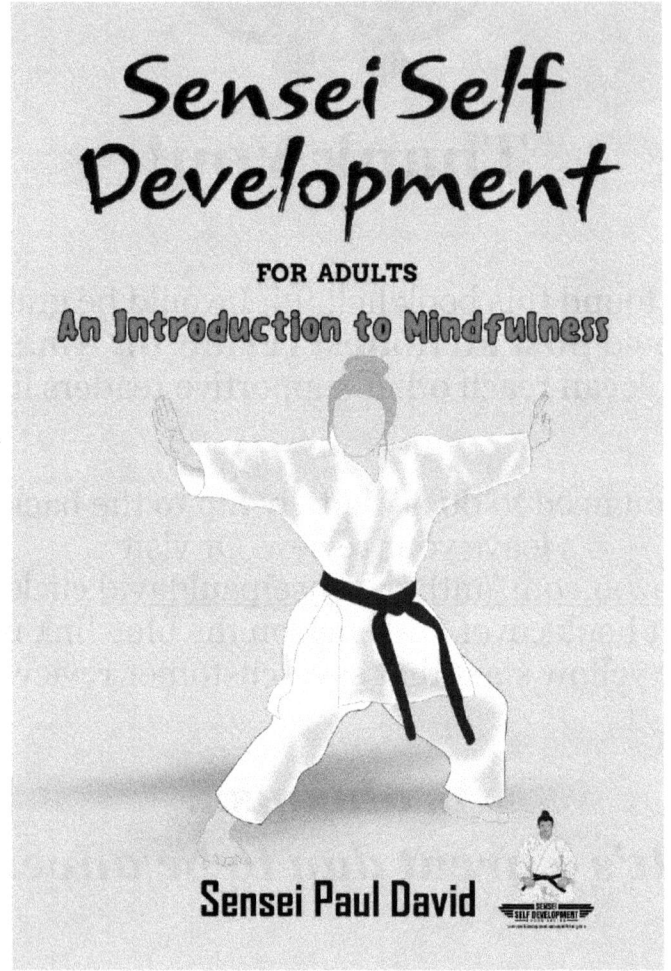

# Check Out The SSD Chronicles Series CLICK HERE

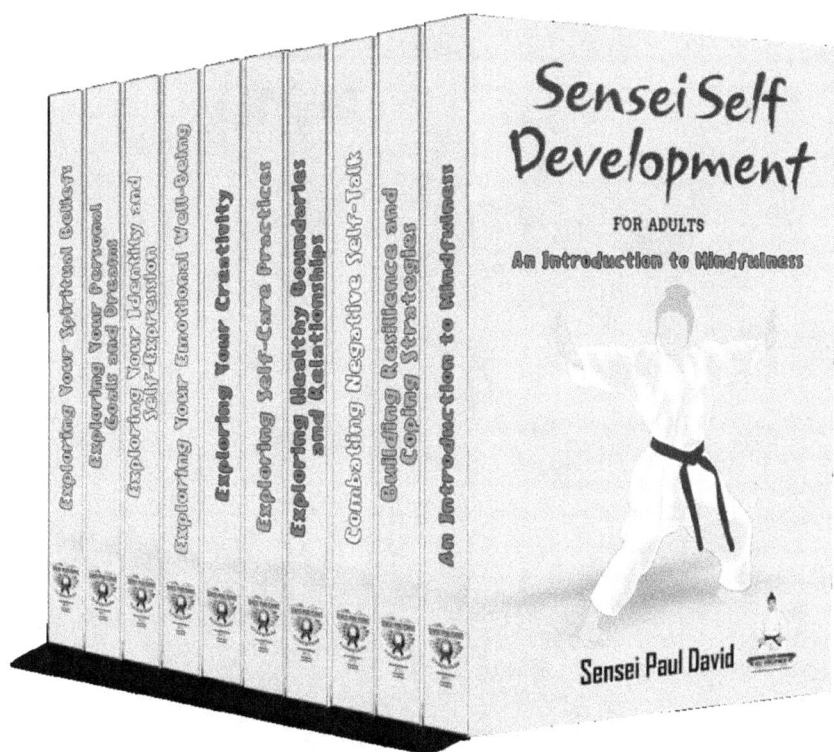

# Get/Share Your FREE All-Ages Mental Health eBook Now at
www.senseiselfdevelopment.com
## Or CLICK HERE

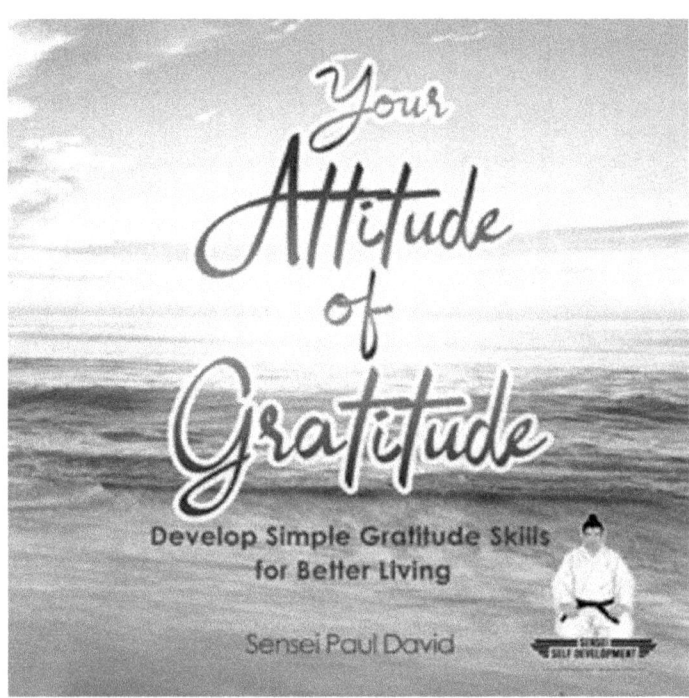

senseiselfdevelopment.com

# Click Another Book In The SSD BOOK SERIES:
senseipublishing.com/SSD_SERIES
## CLICK HERE

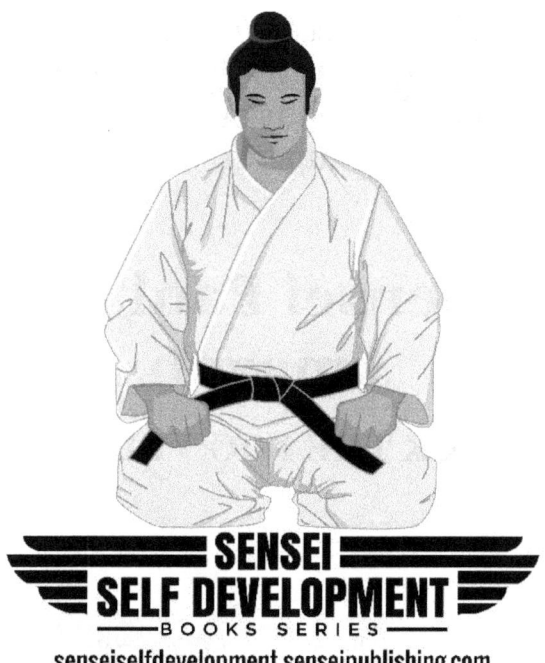

# Join Our Publishing Journey!

If you would like to receive FREE BOOKS, please visit **www.senseipublishing.com**. Join our newsletter by entering your email address in the pop-up box

# Follow Sensei Paul David on Amazon

### CLICK THE LOGO BELOW

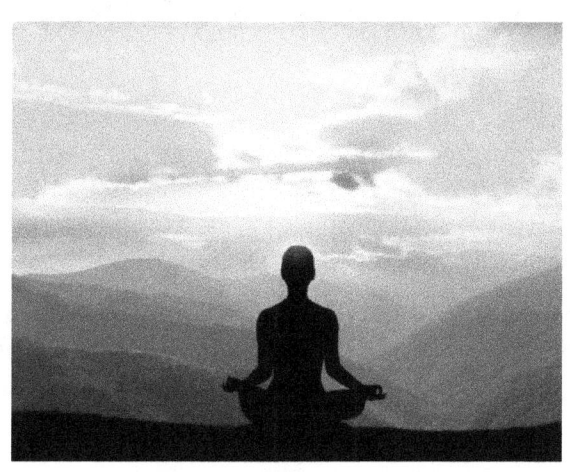

## FREE BONUS!!!
## Experience Over 25 FREE Engaging Guided Meditations!

Prized Skills & Practices for Adults & Kids. Help Restore Deep-Sleep, Lower Stress, Improve Posture, Navigate Uncertainty & More.

Download the Free Insight Timer App and click the link below:
**http://insig.ht/sensei_paul**

# About Sensei Publishing

Sensei Publishing commits itself to helping people of all ages transform into better versions of themselves by providing high-quality and research-based self-development books with an emphasis on mental health and guided meditations. Sensei Publishing offers well-written e-books, audiobooks, paperbacks and online courses that simplify complicated but practical topics in line with its mission to inspire people towards positive transformation.

It's a great day to be alive!

# About the Author

I create simple & transformative eBooks & Guided Meditations for Adults & Children proven to help navigate uncertainty, solve niche problems & bring families closer together.

I'm a former finance project manager, private pilot, jiu-jitsu instructor, musician & former University of Toronto Fitness Trainer. I prefer a science-based approach to focus on these & other areas in my life to stay humble & hungry to evolve. I hope you enjoy my work and I'd love to hear your feedback.

- It's a great day to be alive!

Sensei Paul David

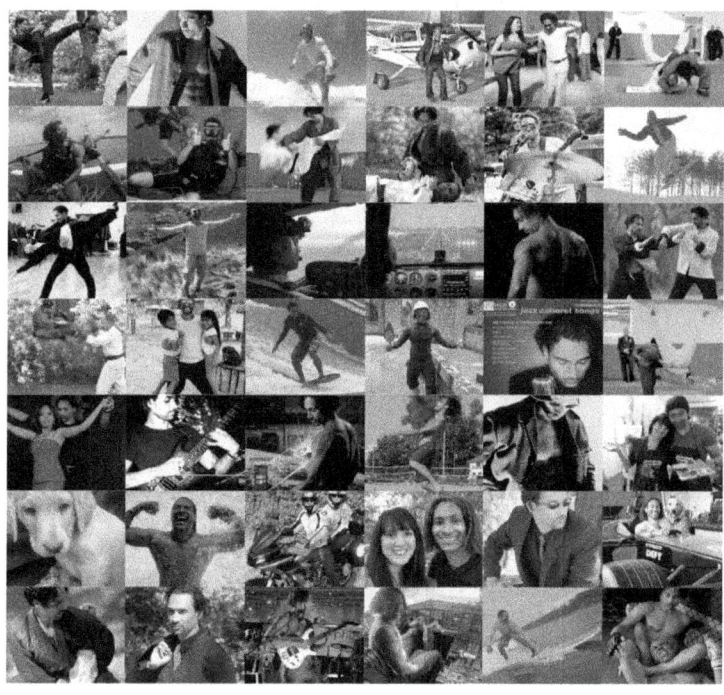

Scan & Follow/Like/Subscribe: Facebook, Instagram, YouTube: @senseipublishing

Scan using your phone/iPad camera for Social Media Visit us at www.senseipublishing.com and sign up for our newsletter to learn more about our exciting books and to experience our FREE Guided Meditations for Kids & Adults.

www.ingramcontent.com/pod-product-compliance
Lightning Source LLC
Chambersburg PA
CBHW070033040426
42333CB00040B/1618